BLOOD TYPE
COOKBOOK

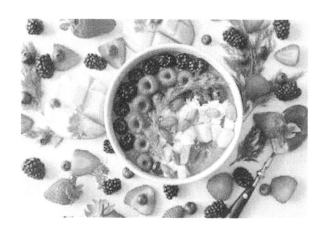

40 ultimate list of healthy, nutritious diet recipes to eat right for your supplements type

ALVIN LEWIS

COPYRIGHT © 2023 BY ALVIN LEWIS

The views and opinions expressed in this book are solely those of the author. The author has made every reasonable effort to ensure that the information provided in this book is accurate and up to date at the time of publication.

TABLE OF CONTENTS

INTRODUCTION

There was a man named Daniel who lived in a busy metropolis. He was just a regular guy who worked long hours at a desk job, ate fast food for lunch, and spent his evenings binge-watching TV shows. He was never very energetic and by no means a health enthusiast. Daniel knew he needed to change, but he didn't know where to begin after his doctor had alerted him to his unhealthy lifestyle.

Daniel discovered a book named "The B Positive Diet Cookbook" one beautiful afternoon while perusing a neighborhood bookstore. He snatched it up and began leafing through the pages, drawn in by the cover's vibrant colors and intriguing title.

A novel idea—a diet specific to an individual's blood type—was discussed in the book. Daniel was positive for blood type B, and the book promised to change his life by enlightening him about the specific nutritional requirements that his body required.

After deciding to buy the book, he couldn't put it down once he started reading it that evening. The book offered comprehensive meal plans, recipes, and advice on how to maximize one's health according to blood type. It was jam-packed with fascinating information regarding the connection between blood type and diet.

Daniel became fully absorbed in the B Positive Diet throughout the course of the following few weeks. He started by cleaning out her pantry, bidding farewell to processed foods and items that were not compatible with her blood type.

Armed with a shopping list tailored to her new diet, he ventured into the grocery store, eager to explore the world of B-positive-friendly foods. He tidied his kitchen, bringing in fresh produce, lean meats, nutritious grains, and fruits in place of processed items. He began preparing his own meals using the book's recipes. Daniel was committed to changing his fast-food habits, even though it was a big shift.

Daniel's body started reacting well to his new diet as the weeks stretched into months. Throughout the day, he felt more energized, and his ability to focus at work increased. His spirits rose, and he became more positive about life in general. He felt as though a veil had parted, allowing him to scc the world in all its vivid hues.

As advised by the book, Daniel also began to include regular exercise in his routine. He started with easy strolls in the park and worked his way up to increasingly difficult exercises. He became more fit overall and began to lose the extra weight that had been bothering him for years.

The improvement in his social life that resulted from his journey was among its most unexpected consequences. Daniel started experimenting with new foods, visiting various eateries, and even enrolling in cooking classes as he grew more mindful of his diet. He discovered that by sharing his newfound enthusiasm with friends and family, he was encouraging them to make better decisions as well.

After a few months became a year, Daniel went to his doctor for a usual checkup and saw remarkable improvements. He no longer met the criteria for pre-diabetes, his blood pressure was normal, and his cholesterol had dramatically decreased. His physician requested to know his secret after being astounded by the change.

Daniel grinned and gave his doctor the B Positive Diet Cookbook; both of them were in awe. They both came to see how information and willpower can transform someone's life for the better.

Daniel's experience with the B Positive Diet enhanced not just his physical but also his mental and emotional state of being. He had found a network of friends who were as committed to leading a better lifestyle as he was, and he had developed a newfound joy for life and cooking. Daniel's life was reviving day by day because of a fortuitous encounter with a book that changed his course.

Understanding Blood Type B-Positive

An essential part of the human body, blood is essential to the preservation of our general well-being. There are various blood types, and each has special qualities and attributes of its own. B-positive (B+) is one of these blood types, and it has a unique set of characteristics. We'll go into great detail about blood type B-positive in this book, covering its traits, compatibility, possible health risks, and lifestyle suggestions.

Blood Type Compatibility:

Comprehending blood type compatibility is essential, particularly in relation to organ transplants or blood transfusions. Red blood cells can be donated by people with B-positive blood to recipients who are B-positive and AB-positive. They can also accept blood from donors who test positive for B and O antibodies. Being aware of your blood type can help save lives in emergency situations by ensuring that the appropriate blood is given.

Health-related Aspects:

Although blood type does not determine one's overall health, some research has looked into possible links between blood types and a person's vulnerability to particular illnesses. Individuals who have B-positive blood may be more vulnerable to certain health issues, like:

1. Increased Infection Risk: According to some study, people with B-positive blood may be more prone to developing specific illnesses. However, a number of factors, such as genetics and lifestyle, affect this risk.

2. Increased Risk of Heart Disease: B-positive blood types may be somewhat more likely to develop heart disease, according to some preliminary research. This emphasizes how crucial it is to continue living a heart-healthy lifestyle.

3. Gut Health: According to the Blood Type Diet, those who have B-positive blood should concentrate on eating a diet that promotes optimal gut health, which may help with digestion and general wellbeing.

It's important to remember that there is currently no solid data to support the assertions made about the relationship between blood type and health.

Way of Life Suggestions:
It's important to lead a healthy lifestyle regardless of your blood type. However, the following lifestyle suggestions will be helpful for people with B-positive blood:

1. Balanced Diet: Consume dairy products, green veggies, lean proteins, and a variety of other foods in a well-rounded diet. Steer clear of red meat overindulgence, even if it's frequently advised for other blood types.

2. Frequent Exercise: To promote heart health and general well-being, partake in regular physical activity.

3. Stress management: Just like everyone else, B-positive people should concentrate on stress-reduction methods including yoga, meditation, and deep breathing exercises.

4. Frequent Check-ups: In order to identify and manage any possible health issues, routine medical check-ups are crucial.

Knowing your blood type—for example, B-positive—can help you make informed decisions about your health, including whether to get a blood transfusion and what foods to eat. But it's crucial to keep in mind that a variety of things affect each person's health; blood type is only one piece of the picture. For individualized health advice and recommendations, always seek the guidance of a healthcare expert.

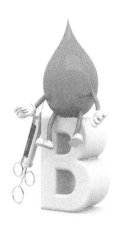

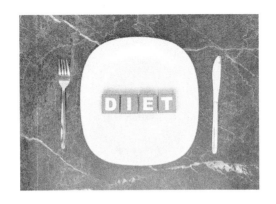

CHAPTER ONE

Blood Type B-Positive Basics

One of the various blood types that people might have is blood type B-positive (B+). For medical needs, such as blood transfusions, organ transplants, and potential dietary concerns, it is imperative to comprehend the basics of this blood type. The following are important fundamentals about blood type B-positive:

1. Antigens: Red blood cells of blood type B-positive have two distinct antigens on their surface: Rh factor (Rhesus factor) and B antigen.
In the name of the blood type, the B antigen determines the "B" and the Rh factor makes it "positive." The blood type is known as B-negative if the Rh factor is missing.

2. Compatibility of Blood: Red blood cells can be donated by B-positive people to B-positive and AB-positive people.

Both B-positive and O-positive donors can give them blood. For blood transfusions to be both safe and successful, compatibility is essential.

3. Adaptability: Because B-positive blood is thought to be very adaptable, it is useful in medical situations and emergencies where certain blood types are hard to come by.

4. Associations for Health: Studies have indicated possible links between blood kinds and health issues. It's important to keep in mind that while B-positive people may be slightly more likely to get certain infections and heart disease, these correlations are not conclusive.

5. Blood Type Diet: people with various blood types ought to adhere to meals that are appropriate to their blood type. This diet usually suggests a balance of lean proteins, green vegetables, and some dairy items for people who test positive for B-chromosome disorders.

6. Theoretically, personality traits: According to certain blood type personality theory proponents, those who have B-positive blood may be creative, flexible, and adaptive. But this notion is unsupported by science, therefore it should be viewed with caution.

7. Genetic Transmission: Genetics determines your blood type; one blood type allele is contributed by each parent. Parents having blood types B, AB, or O can pass on blood type B to their offspring.

Knowing your blood type—for example, B-positive—is important for dietary and medicinal decisions. Blood type should not be the only factor in determining your lifestyle choices, even while it may influence some aspects of food and health. Always seek the advice of medical specialists for specific advice, and keep in mind that many factors other than blood type can affect your general well-being.

Characteristics of B-Positive Individuals

Blood type B-positive (B+) is one of the several blood types, and some people believe that our blood type can influence our personality traits and behaviors. While scientific research has not provided conclusive evidence for the blood type personality theory, some proponents suggest that individuals with B-positive blood may exhibit certain characteristics. It's important to note that these characteristics are based on anecdotal evidence and should be taken with caution. Here are some commonly attributed traits to B-positive individuals:

1. Flexibility: B-positive individuals are often described as adaptable and flexible. They tend to

handle change well and can adjust to new situations and environments with ease. This adaptability can be an asset in a variety of life circumstances.

2. Creativity: Creativity is another trait often associated with B-positive individuals. They may have a natural flair for artistic endeavors and problem-solving, allowing them to approach challenges with innovative solutions.

3. Sociable: People with B-positive blood are thought to be outgoing and sociable. They tend to enjoy social interactions, make friends easily, and have a wide circle of acquaintances. This can make them natural networkers.

4. Optimism: B-positive individuals are often believed to have an optimistic outlook on life. They tend to see the silver lining in situations and maintain a positive attitude even in challenging times.

5. Ambitious: B-positive individuals are said to be goal-oriented and ambitious. They set high standards for themselves and work diligently to achieve their objectives. This drive can lead to success in various aspects of life.

6. Independent Thinkers: B-positive individuals may exhibit independent thinking and a willingness to question the status quo. They tend to form their opinions after careful consideration and research.

7. Tolerance: B-positive individuals are thought to be open-minded and accepting of different perspectives and beliefs. They typically have a high level of tolerance for diversity and may be more accommodating in their interactions.

8. Emotional Sensitivity: Some proponents of the blood type personality theory suggest that B-positive individuals can be emotionally sensitive. They may empathize with others and respond to emotional cues more readily.

It's important to reiterate that the blood type personality theory lacks scientific credibility. The idea that blood type can determine personality traits is not supported by scientific research or consensus. Our personalities are influenced by a complex interplay of genetic, environmental, and social factors. While blood type may have some minor biological implications, it should not be considered a definitive determinant of one's character.

People are unique individuals, and their personalities cannot be reduced to a single characteristic based solely on their blood type. It's essential to approach discussions of personality with an open and critical mindset, considering multiple factors that contribute to our diverse and multifaceted human nature.

Don't wait – start your "Deliciously B-Positive" culinary adventure today!

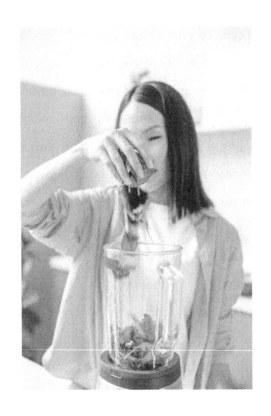

CHAPTER TWO

Nutrient-Rich Foods for B-Positives

Embracing the Blood Type B Positive diet opens up a world of nutrient-rich foods that can help you maintain your well-being. While this diet approach is a personal journey that might not be universally accepted, many individuals find it beneficial to include nutrient-dense options in their daily meals. Here are some nutrient-rich foods that can support your journey to better health

Protein Sources for B-Positives

Blood type B-positive people have a particular nutritional profile that can improve their overall health and wellbeing. Blood type B individuals should eat a balanced diet that includes a variety of food groups, such as lean proteins, fruits, vegetables, and grains. However, it's crucial to concentrate on protein sources that are suitable for this blood type.

The following protein sources are appropriate for people with B-positive blood type:

1. Lean Meats: Skinless chicken, turkey, and game meats like deer are examples of lean meats that are thought to be healthy choices for those with blood type B. These meats can play a significant role in a balanced diet because they are high in protein.

2. Fish: For those with blood type B, a variety of fish species are great providers of protein. In addition to being high in protein, fish like salmon, trout, mackerel, and halibut also contain important omega-3 fatty acids that can promote heart and brain health.

3. Dairy Products: Blood type B individuals can include moderate amounts of dairy products in their

diet. Choose low-fat or fat-free products such as cheese, kefir, and yogurt. For gut health, these dairy products can include probiotics, calcium, and protein.

4. Eggs: Suitable for a wide range of recipes, eggs are a flexible source of protein. They are also a good source of vitamins, minerals, and essential amino acids that are vital for good health.

5. Plant-Based Proteins: Although it is typically recommended that people with blood type B eat animal-based proteins, for diversity and extra fiber, plant-based choices such as seitan, tofu, tempeh, and legumes (lentils, black beans, and chickpeas) can be included in the diet.

6. Nuts and Seeds: For those with blood type B, nuts and seeds including chia seeds, walnuts, and almonds are excellent sources of protein. Additionally, they are high in fiber and good fats, which support satiety and energy maintenance.

It is crucial to bear in mind that the Blood Type Diet is a nutritional idea that has generated some controversy and that there is scant scientific data to support its efficacy. Regardless of blood type, a well-balanced diet with a range of protein sources can improve general health.

Fruits and Vegetables for Optimal Health

Many people want to be as healthy as possible, and eating right is a big part of that. The Blood Type Diet recommends that several fruits and vegetables can be especially helpful for people who have a B-positive blood type. Despite its detractors and scant scientific backing, a diet heavy in fruits and vegetables is beneficial for people of all blood types. This in-depth guide examines the significance of fruits and vegetables for people with blood type B-positive and provides a plethora of options to help you optimize your diet for general health.

1. Berries: Antioxidants, which are vital for optimal health, are abundant in blueberries, strawberries, raspberries, and blackberries. They offer taste and nutrition to your diet and are thought to be suitable with blood type B.

2. Plums: Because of their apparent compatibility, plums are frequently advised for those with blood type B. They are an excellent source of fiber and vitamins.

3. Pineapples: Known for their digestive enzyme, bromelain, pineapples are a tropical fruit. They may help with digestion and make a tasty addition to your diet.

4. Apples: A versatile and healthful snack choice, apples are juicy and crisp. They are an excellent source of vital vitamins and fiber.

5. Papaya: A tropical fruit that can improve your general health, papaya is rich in vitamins, minerals, and digestive enzymes.

Vegetables for People with Blood Type B:

1. Green Leafy Vegetables: Make sure your diet is rich in broccoli, kale, and spinach. They are abundant in fiber, which promotes digestive health, and vitamins A and C.

2. Bell Peppers: Rich in vitamins and antioxidants, red, green, and yellow bell peppers give your food color and taste.

3. Carrots: Carrots are a versatile and nutrient-dense vegetable. They are a delicious complement to salads, the ideal snack, and a base for many other recipes.

4. Eggplant: A versatile vegetable that may be roasted, grilled, or added to stir-fries, eggplant is frequently advised for those with blood type B.

5. Green and red cabbage are great options for incorporating crunch and nutrition into your food. Because of its high vitamin and mineral content, cabbage is a great complement to any diet.

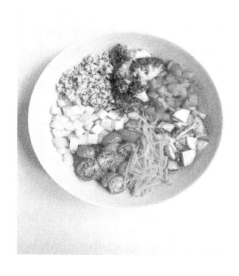

B-Positive Whole Grains and Carbohydrates

A balanced diet must include whole grains and carbs since they provide energy, fiber, and a variety of nutrients. The Blood Type Diet recommends certain whole grains and carbohydrates that may be especially helpful for people who have blood type B. Even though there isn't much scientific proof to back up the Blood Type Diet, eating more of these whole grains and carbohydrates can improve your health in general.

Whole Grains for People with Blood Type B:

1. Brown Rice: Packed with fiber, vitamins, and minerals, brown rice is an incredibly nourishing whole grain. It is a common ingredient in many different types of cooking, including stir-fries and grain bowls.

2. Oats: Rich in soluble fiber, oats can help control blood sugar levels and strengthen heart health. You can eat them as oatmeal, use them in smoothies, or include them into baking creations.

3. Quinoa: Quinoa has all nine of the essential amino acids, making it a complete protein. It's also a popular option for people with dietary requirements because it's strong in fiber and gluten-free.

4. Millet: An ancient grain free of gluten, millet is high in antioxidants, phosphorus, and magnesium. It goes well with salads, side dishes, and porridges.

5. Buckwheat: Although it sounds similar to wheat, buckwheat is inherently gluten-free. It's an excellent source of fiber, protein, and other nutrients. Pancakes, noodles, and other baked items can be made with buckwheat flour.

B-Positive Blood Type: Carbohydrates

potatoes are a nutrient-dense carbohydrate that's high in fiber, vitamins, and minerals. They are a better option for blood sugar control because they have a lower glycemic index than normal potatoes.

Brown rice and other healthy grains can be used to make rice cakes, which are a quick and wholesome snack choice. For extra taste and nutrients, you may top them with hummus, avocado, or nut butter.

Legumes: Legumes are great providers of fiber, protein, and carbs. Examples of legumes are lentils, chickpeas, and black beans. They can be used to make plant-based burgers and dips, as well as added to soups, stews, and salads.

Whole Grain Pasta: Rather than consuming refined pasta, choose whole grain or pasta made from legumes. These choices offer more minerals and fiber, which improves digestion and general health.

Fruits: Fruits are a good source of fiber, vitamins, and carbohydrates in addition to their inherent sugar content. For a well-rounded nutrient intake, include a range of fruits in your diet, including berries, apples, bananas, and oranges.

Along with a range of other nutrient-dense foods, including whole grains and carbohydrates in your diet can help with digestion, energy levels, and general well-being. Keep in mind that every person has a different reaction to food, so it's important to figure out what suits your body the best and seek the counsel of medical professionals for specific recommendations.

Healthy Fats for B-Positive Individuals

The proper kinds of fats can be very important in maintaining general health for those with a B-positive blood type. An appropriate diet must include fats. Though the Blood Type Diet offers recommendations for food choices, it's vital to keep in mind that there isn't much scientific evidence to support this diet. However, adding healthy fats to your diet has a number of advantages for your health. B-positive Blood Type-Friendly Fats includes:

Extra virgin olive oil is widely regarded as heart-healthy and is a mainstay of the Mediterranean diet. It contains a lot of monounsaturated fats, which may lower the risk of inflammation and heart disease. Use for salad dressings, sautéing, or drizzling over cooked food.

Avocado: A special fruit, avocados are incredibly abundant in heart-healthy monounsaturated fats. In addition, it offers several vitamins, fiber, potassium, and other necessary elements. Savor avocado slices on salads, toast, or as a foundation for creamy dressings and sauces.

Nuts: Rich sources of monounsaturated and polyunsaturated fats, nuts such as cashews, walnuts, and almonds are healthy fats. They also contain a lot of fiber, protein, and several vitamins and minerals. Snacking on a tiny handful of nuts is a filling and healthy treat.

Seeds: Rich in omega-3 fatty acids, chia, flax, and pumpkin seeds are among the seeds that are filled with healthful fats. The heart and brain are supported by these lipids. They go well with yogurt and smoothies, as well as salads.

Omega-3 fatty acids, which are abundant in fatty fish like salmon, mackerel, and trout and have anti-inflammatory qualities, are vital for cardiovascular health. Make it a point to frequently eat these fish.

Coconut: Although it contains medium-chain triglycerides (MCTs), which are good for energy and brain function, coconuts come in a variety of forms, including oil, shredded coconut, and milk. Use coconut milk in recipes or as a substitute for oil when cooking.

Natural nut butters such as peanut butter and almond butter offer a source of good fats.

Benefits of Eating According to Your Blood Type

This cookbook for Blood Type B Positives explores the fascinating idea of customizing your diet to your specific blood type. Although the Blood Type Diet's scientific foundation is still up for debate, there are some possible benefits to this strategy that you might find intriguing:

1. Improved Digestion: Eating according to your blood type can help with better digestion. A diet high in lean meats and green vegetables is often beneficial for blood type B persons since it can help improve gut health.

2. Enhanced Energy: You may experience an increase in energy by tailoring your diet to your blood type. You may help your body work at its best

and feel more alive by putting an emphasis on foods that are suitable with your blood type.

3. **Potential Weight Management:** Some people say that following the dietary guidelines according to their blood type has assisted them in reaching and maintaining a healthy weight. They may have less cravings and better control over their weight if they stay away from foods that are less suitable with their blood type.

4. **Optimal Nutrient Absorption:** You may maximize the absorption of nutrients by customizing your diet to match your blood type. This guarantees that the meals you eat are providing you with the maximum amount of health and wellness.

5. **Individualized Approach:** Customization is key to the Blood Type Diet. It inspires you to pay attention to how your body reacts to various meals and modify your diet accordingly. With this method,

you can customize your diet to meet your specific requirements and tastes.

6. Investigating Healthier Options: Adopting a Blood Type Diet frequently prompts people to look into healthier ingredients and preparation techniques. Your concentration on complete, unprocessed foods may cause you to incline toward a diet that is more balanced and nutrient-dense by nature.

Although there is disagreement regarding the Blood Type Diet's scientific validity, it may be beneficial to pay attention to your body's individual signals and nutritional requirements. Keep an open mind as you work through the recipes in this cookbook and discover how matching your diet to your blood type can improve your overall health.

CHAPTER THREE

Recipes for a B-Positive Lifestyle

The significance of nutrition in achieving a well-rounded and robust lifestyle cannot be emphasized. A person's food is a major factor in determining their general health and wellbeing. This cookbook denotes a gastronomic strategy designed to support and maintain a blood type B-positive (B+) state.

This note will explore the idea of eating in accordance with one's blood type, specifically for those who are blood type B+, and offer advice on how to create a diet that supports this idea.

Breakfast Ideas Recipes

Avocado toast with poached egg

Ingredients:

- One piece of bread, whole-grain
- One juicy avocado
- One egg
- Add pepper and salt to taste.
- Flakes of red pepper (optional)

Preparations:

The whole-grain bread is toasted. Spread the mashed, ripe avocado over the toast. Poach the egg to your desired level of doneness. Place the poached egg on top of the avocado toast. If preferred, add red pepper flakes, salt, and pepper for seasoning.

Prep Time: 15 minutes

Smoothie with Berries and Almond Butter

Ingredients:

- one cup of blueberries, raspberries, and strawberries combined
- One banana
- One tablespoon of almond butter

- Almond milk, one cup
- One teaspoon honey, if desired

Preparations:

In a blender, combine all the ingredients. Mix until homogeneous. If desired, add honey after tasting.

Prep Time: Five minutes to prepare

Parfait with Greek Yogurt

Ingredients:

- Greek yogurt, one cup
- One-half cup granola
- Mixture of 1/2 cup berries (strawberries, raspberries, and blueberries)
- One tablespoon of honey

Preparations:

In a glass or bowl, arrange Greek yogurt, granola, and mixed berries. Pour some honey on it.

Prep Time:5 minutes

Tofu Stir-fried with Tomatoes and Spinach

Ingredients:

- 1/2 cup of firm tofu crumbles
- 1/2 cup of fresh spinach

- 1/2 cup of tomatoes, diced
- 1/4 teaspoon turmeric
- Add pepper and salt to taste.

Preparations:

Crumble the tofu and cook it in a pan until it begins to brown. Cook the spinach until it wilts by adding the tomatoes and spinach. Use pepper, salt, and turmeric for seasoning.

Prep Time: 10 minutes.

Pancakes with peanut butter and banana

Ingredients:

- Half a cup of whole wheat pancake mixture
- half a cup of almond milk
- one mashed, ripe banana
- Two teaspoon organic peanut butter

Preparations:

In a bowl, combine together pancake mix and almond milk. Add the mashed banana and stir. Pancakes are cooked on a griddle. Drizzle with natural peanut butter before serving.

Prep Time: 20 minutes

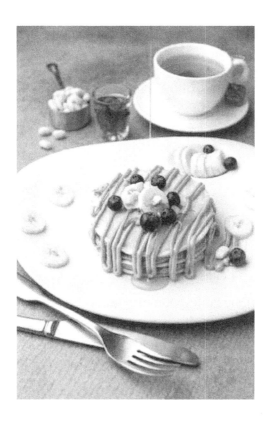

Cream cheese and smoked salmon wrap

Ingredients:

- One entire-grain wrap
- Two tablespoon cream cheese
- Two pieces of salmon smoked
- 1/4 cup of cucumbers, cut up
- 1/4 cup of greens, mixed

Preparations:

Spread the whole-grain wrapper with cream cheese. Place cucumber, mixed greens, and smoked salmon in layers. After rolling, cut it in half.

Prep Time: 10 minutes

Breakfast Bowl with Quinoa

Ingredients:

- 50 ml of cooked quinoa
- 1/2 cup Greek yogurt
- 1/4 cup of berry mixture
- One tablespoon of honey
- One tablespoon of finely chopped nuts (walnuts, almonds, etc.)

Preparations:

Add Greek yogurt and quinoa to a bowl. Add chopped nuts, honey, and mixed berries on top.

Prep Time: 10 minutes

Veggies Omelet

Ingredients:

- Two eggs
- 1/4 cup of bell peppers, chopped

- Diced tomatoes, 1/4 cup
- 1/4 cup of onions, chopped
- 1/4 cup of spinach, chopped
- Add pepper and salt to taste.

Preparations:

In a bowl, whisk the eggs. While the skillet is hot, sauté the vegetables until they become soft. Cover the veggies with the eggs, then simmer until they are set. Once folded, serve.

Prep Time: 15 minutes

Almond and Apple Overnight Oats

Ingredients:

- Oats, half a cup rolled
- Almond milk, one cup
- 1½ apples, chopped
- One teaspoon almond butter
- One teaspoon honey

Preparations:

In a jar, mix almond milk with rolled oats. Add the honey, almond butter, and sliced apple. Give it a good stir, cover, and chill for the night.

Prep Time:Five minutes *(including an overnight soak)*

Spinach and Mushrooms Breakfast Burrito

Ingredients:

- Two eggs
- Sliced mushrooms, half a cup
- half a cup of spinach, chopped
- A single whole grain tortilla
- Add pepper and salt to taste.

Preparations:

In a pan, scramble the eggs. Cook the spinach and mushrooms by sautéing them. Spoon the spinach, mushrooms, and scrambled eggs into the whole-grain tortilla. Add pepper and salt for seasoning. After rolling, serve the tortilla.

Prep Time:15 minutes

These breakfast recipes for B-positive people are full of nutrients and provide a range of options, from savory to sweet, to help you start the day right. Maintain a balanced and health-conscious diet while indulging in your tasty and nourishing breakfast.

Satisfying Lunches

Quinoa bowl and Grilled Chicken

Ingredients:

- 1 cup of quinoa, cooked
- 6 ounces of grilled, sliced chicken breast
- Steamed broccoli, half a cup
- Sliced red bell peppers, half a cup
- Two teaspoon of olive oil
- One-third cup lemon juice

Add pepper and salt to taste.

Instructions:

Follow the directions on the package to cook the quinoa. After the chicken is cooked through, slice it. Steam broccoli for a soft texture. Quinoa, broccoli, grilled chicken, and sliced red bell peppers should all be combined in a bowl. Pour in some lemon juice and olive oil. Add salt to taste and pepper for seasoning.

Stir-fried Lentil and Vegetables

Ingredients:

- 1 cup of lentils, cooked

- One cup of mixed veggies, such as carrots, snap peas, and bell peppers
- Two teaspoon of soy sauce (low sodium)
- One teaspoon of sesame oil
- one minced garlic clove
- One teaspoon freshly grated ginger

Instructions:

As directed on the package, prepare the lentils. Sesame oil is heated in a pan. Add the grated ginger and minced garlic, and cook for one minute. Stir-fry the mixed vegetables until they become soft. Add the soy sauce and cooked lentils, then fully heat. Warm up the food.

Stir-fried Turkey with Vegetables

Ingredients:

- 1 pound of turkey meat
- 1 cup of mixed veggies, including bell peppers, broccoli, and zucchini
- One teaspoon of olive oil
- Two teaspoon of soy sauce (low sodium)
- One teaspoon honey
- One teaspoon finely chopped, fresh ginger

Instructions:

Warm up some olive oil in a pan and add the ground turkey. Stir-fry the mixed vegetables until they become soft. Combine the ginger, honey, and soy sauce in a small bowl. Stir thoroughly after adding the sauce to the turkey and veggies. Simmer for a few more minutes, or until well heated. Serve with quinoa or brown rice.

Lemon and Herb Baked Salmon

Ingredients:

- 2 filets of salmon
- Two teaspoon of olive oil
- 1 sliced lemon
- Two minced garlic cloves
- Fresh herbs, such as thyme and rosemary
- Add pepper and salt to taste.

Instructions:

Turn the oven on to 375°F, or 190°C. The salmon fillets should be put on a baking pan. Add a drizzle of olive oil and top with minced garlic. Arrange fresh herbs and lemon slices on top of the salmon. Add pepper and salt for seasoning. Bake the salmon for 15 to 20 minutes, or until it is well done. Accompany with a crisp salad or a dish of steaming veggies.

Salad with Quinoa and Black Beans

Instructions:

- 1 cup of quinoa, cooked
- One cup of cooked or canned black beans, rinsed, drained, and
- 50 ml of corn kernels
- half a cup of tomatoes, diced
- 1/4 cup of freshly chopped cilantro
- Two tablespoons of olive oil and one juiced lime
- To taste, add salt and pepper.

Preparations:

Quinoa, black beans, corn, diced tomatoes, and chopped cilantro should all be combined in a big bowl. Mix the olive oil and lime juice in a small bowl. After adding the dressing to the salad, toss to mix. Add salt to taste and pepper for seasoning. Served chilled.

Stir-fried Shrimp with Asparagus

Ingredients:

- One pound of big, peeled and deveined shrimp
- One bundle of asparagus, pruned and divided into segments
- Two minced garlic cloves
- One teaspoon of olive oil
- Two teaspoon of soy sauce (low sodium)
- One teaspoon honey
- one-half teaspoon freshly grated ginger

Instructions:

Shrimp should be stir-fried in hot olive oil until they turn pink and are done. When the asparagus is crisp-tender, add the minced garlic and simmer. Combine the ginger, honey, and soy sauce in a small bowl. Stir thoroughly after adding the sauce to the shrimp and asparagus. Simmer a few minutes longer. Serve over quinoa or brown rice.

Ground turkey and stuffed bell peppers

Ingredients:

- Four peppers

- 1 cup cooked brown rice
- 1 pound ground turkey
- 1 cup chopped tomatoes
- Diced Onions, 1/2 cup
- 1/2 cup washed, drained, and cooked black beans (from can).
- Half a cup of mozzarella cheese, shredded
- Add pepper and salt to taste.

Instructions:

Turn the oven on to 375°F, or 190°C. Slice off the bell peppers' tops, then take out the seeds and membranes. The ground turkey should be browned in a big skillet. Cook the onions until they become tender. Add the cooked rice, black beans, and diced tomatoes and stir. Add pepper and salt for seasoning. Stuff the turkey and rice mixture into the bell peppers. Stuffed peppers should be baked for 25 to 30 minutes, or until they arc soft, in a baking dish. After adding a sprinkle of mozzarella cheese, bake for a further five minutes, or until the cheese has melted. Warm up the food.

Spinach and mushrooms Omelet

Ingredients:

- Two eggs
- Half a cup of spinach, chopped
- 1/4 cup of mushrooms, sliced
- Diced tomatoes, 1/4 cup
- 1/4 cup of onions, chopped
- Two teaspoon of olive oil
- To taste, add salt and pepper.

Instructions:

In a nonstick pan, warm up some olive oil. Add the mushrooms and onions and sauté until they begin to brown. Cook the spinach until it wilts by adding it along with the diced tomatoes. Whisk the eggs, pepper, and salt together in a bowl. Cover the veggies with the egg mixture and simmer until it sets. After folding, serve the omelette in half.

Honey-Lime Dressing with Fruit Salad

Ingredients:

- Various fruits (including oranges, kiwis, pineapple, and berries)

- Two teaspoon of honey
- 1 lime's juice
- Garnish with fresh mint leaves

Instructions:

As needed, wash, peel, and chop the fruits. To make the dressing, combine lime juice and honey in a small bowl. Pour the dressing over the mixed fruit. Add some mint leaves as a garnish. Serve cold.

Pesto-Crusted Zucchini Noodles

Ingredients:

- Twirled two medium zucchinis into noodles
- one-fourth cup pesto basilico
- Grated cherry tomatoes, cut in half
- Add pepper and salt to taste.

Instructions:

With the use of a vegetable peeler or spiralizer, create noodles out of the zucchini. Heat a small amount of olive oil in a big skillet over medium heat When the zucchini noodles are soft but still crisp, add them and sauté for two to three minutes. Stir in the chopped cherry tomatoes and pesto sauce. Cook the mixture for a further two to three minutes, or until well heated. Add salt to taste and pepper for seasoning. Sprinkle some grated Parmesan cheese over the zucchini noodles before serving.

These blood type B recipes provide a range of tasty and healthy options, from vegetable-focused meals to protein-rich ones. Savor these meals as a part of a diet that is well-balanced and tailored to your individual blood type and nutritional needs.

Dinner Recipes

Steamed Asparagus And Quinoa With Grilled Salmon

Components:
- 2 fillets of salmon
- One-cup quinoa
- One bunch of green beans
- Two teaspoon of olive oil
- Juiced one lime
- Add pepper and salt to taste.

Instructions:

Set the oven or grill to a medium-high temperature. Salmon fillets are seasoned with salt, pepper, lemon juice, and olive oil. The salmon should flake easily with a fork after 8 to 10 minutes on each side under the grill or in the oven. In the meantime, prepare the quinoa per the directions on the package. Steam asparagus for crisp-tender results. Arrange the cooked quinoa on a bed of grilled salmon, and accompany it with steamed asparagus.

Tofu With Mixed Vegetables Stir-fried

Components:

- One cubed block of extra-firm tofu
- Two cups of mixed veggies, such as broccoli, snap peas, and bell peppers
- Two teaspoon of olive oil
- Two teaspoon of soy sauce (low sodium)
- One teaspoon honey
- One teaspoon finely chopped, fresh ginger

Instructions:

In a big pan or wok, heat the olive oil. Cubed tofu should be stir-fried till golden brown all throughout.

Stir-fry the mixed vegetables until they become crisp-tender. Combine the ginger, honey, and soy sauce in a small bowl. Stir thoroughly after adding the sauce to the tofu and veggies. Serve with quinoa or brown rice.

Brown Rice And Vegetable Skewers With Chicken

Components:

- Two chicken breasts, skinned and boneless, chopped into pieces
- Various veggies (including cherry tomatoes, zucchini, and bell peppers)
- Two teaspoon of olive oil
- Two teaspoon of lemon juice
- One teaspoon of dehydrated oregano
- Add pepper and salt to taste.
- Cooked brown rice

Instructions:

Warm up the broiler or grill. Put veggies and chicken on skewers. Combine the olive oil, lemon juice, oregano, salt, and pepper in a small bowl. Apply the olive oil mixture to the skewers. For about 15-20 minutes, turning regularly, grill or broil the skewers until the chicken is cooked through and the vegetables are soft. Transfer to warmed brown rice and serve.

Shrimp Sautéed with Garlic and Spinach

Components:

- One pound of big, peeled and deveined shrimp
- two cups of raw spinach.
- three minced garlic cloves
- Two teaspoon of olive oil
- lime juice from one
- To taste, add salt and pepper.

Instructions:

Heat the olive oil in a large skillet. Sauté minced garlic for about 1 minute. Add the shrimp and cook for 2 to 3 minutes on each side, or until they turn pink. Add the fresh spinach and stir, allowing it to wilt. Sprinkle it with salt and pepper and drizzle with lemon juice. Warm up the food.

Stir-fried Turkey with Vegetables

Components:

- 1 pound of turkey meat
- 1 cup of mixed veggies, including bell peppers, broccoli, and zucchini
- Two teaspoon of olive oil
- Two teaspoon of soy sauce (low sodium)
- One teaspoon honey
- One teaspoon finely chopped, fresh ginger

Instructions:

Heat up some olive oil in a big skillet and brown the ground turkey. Stir-fry the mixed vegetables until they become soft. Combine the ginger, honey, and soy sauce in a small bowl. Stir thoroughly after adding the sauce to the turkey and veggies. Simmer for a few more minutes, or until well heated.Serve with quinoa or brown rice.

Chicken Breast Stuffed with Spinach and Mushrooms

Components:

- Two skinless and boneless chicken breasts
- Two cups of raw spinach.

- Sliced mushrooms, half a cup
- Two minced garlic cloves
- Two teaspoon of olive oil
- Add pepper and salt to taste.

Instructions:

Turn the oven on to 375°F, or 190°C. Sliced mushrooms and minced garlic should be cooked in hot olive oil in a skillet until they begin to brown. Add the fresh spinach and stir, allowing it to wilt. Cut a cut to form a pocket in each chicken breast. Place a filling of the spinach and mushroom mixture inside each chicken breast. To seasoning add salt and pepper to the chicken. Bake the chicken for 25 to 30 minutes, or until it is thoroughly done. Warm up the food.

Vegetable and Lentil Soup

Components:

- 1 cup of lentils, dried
- Four cups vegetable broth and one cup of mixed veggies (onions, carrots, and celery)
- Two minced garlic cloves
- Two teaspoon of olive oil

- A single tsp of dried thyme
- Add pepper and salt to taste.

Instructions:

In a big pot, heat the olive oil. Diced onions, minced garlic, and other vegetables should be sautéed until they are tender. After draining and rinsing, add the lentils to the pot. Add the dried thyme, salt, pepper, and vegetable broth and stir. Simmer for about 30-40 minutes, or until the lentils are tender. Serve warm as a hearty soup.

Savor these dinner recipes that suit blood types B-positive. These recipes combine nutritious grains, veggies, and a range of protein sources to create a filling and well-balanced supper.

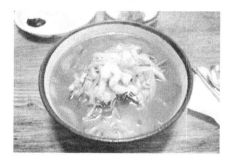

Snacks and Desserts

Rice Cakes With Almond Butter And Bananas

Ingredients:

- Two cakes of brown rice
- Double-stick of almond butter
- One ripe banana, cut.

Instructions:

On each rice cake, spread 1 spoonful of almond butter. Place slices of banana on top. Serve right away.

Prep Time: 5 minutes

Berries and Honey with Greek Yogurt

Ingredients:

- Greek yogurt, one cup
- Mixture of 1/2 cup berries (strawberries, raspberries, and blueberries)
- One tablespoon of honey

Instructions:

Spoon Greek yogurt into a bowl. Add mixed berries on top. Pour some honey on it.

Prep Time: 5 minutes

Almond and Dark Chocolate Clusters

Ingredients:

- 50 milligrams of dark chocolate chips 70% cacao or more
- half a cup of whole almonds
- Sea salt to use as a garnish

Instructions:

In a microwave-safe bowl, melt dark chocolate chips for 20 seconds at a time, stirring in between, until smooth. Add whole almonds and stir until evenly coated. Drop heaping spoonfuls of the mixture onto a tray lined with parchment paper. Add a small amount of sea salt on top. Let it cool and solidify. Savor these crispy almond clusters covered in chocolate.

Prep Time: 15 minutes *(plus cooling time)*

Apple Slices With Almond Butter

Ingredients:

- One sliced apple
- Two teaspoons of almond butter
- *Optional*: sprinkle with cinnamon

Instructions:

Cut the apple into wedges or thin rounds. Dipped in almond butter, dip the apple slices. If desired, top with a cinnamon sprinkle.

Prep Time: 5 minutes

Pears Baked with Cinnamon

Ingredients:

- Two ripe pears, cored and cut in half
- One teaspoon of cinnamon
- Two teaspoon of honey
- 1/4 cup of walnuts, chopped (optional)

Instructions:

Turn the oven on to 375°F, or 190°C. Put the pears cut in half on a baking pan. Drizzle with honey and sprinkle with cinnamon. Bake the pears for 20 to 25 minutes, or until they are soft. If desired, sprinkle chopped walnuts on top.

Prep Time: 30 minutes

Berry and Chia Seed Pudding

Ingredients:

- Three teaspoon of chia seeds
- Almond milk, one cup

- 1/2 cup of mixed berries (raspberries, blueberries, and strawberries)
- One teaspoon honey, if desired

Instructions:

Chia seeds and almond milk should be combined in a container or bowl. Give it a good stir and set aside for a few minutes. After another stir, chill for a minimum of two hours or overnight. If preferred, add a drizzle of honey and top with a mixture of berries.

Prep Time: 5 minutes *(plus cooling time)*

B-positive blood type holders can find a variety of sweet and filling options in these snack and dessert recipes. They are made to be tasty, easy to prepare, and appropriate for a well-balanced diet. As part of your healthy lifestyle, savor these pleasures.

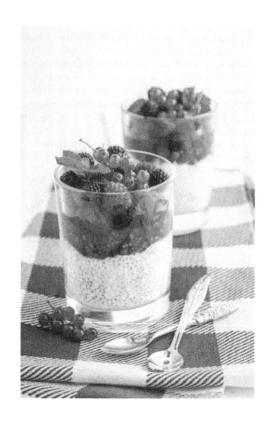

CHAPTER FOUR

Meal Planning and Exercise Fitness Tips

Meal planning is an essential aspect of following any specific dietary guidelines, including the Blood Type Diet for B-positive individuals. This diet suggests that individuals with a B-positive blood type may benefit from certain food choices and restrictions

20-Days Sample Meal plans

DAY 1:

Breakfast:

- Eggs in a scramble with spinach and mushrooms
- Whole-grain toast

Lunch: Mixed greens, bell peppers, and grilled chicken salad dressed with an olive oil vinaigrette

Dinner:

- Salmon baked with quinoa
- Steaming broccoli

DAY 2:

Breakfast: Greek yogurt topped with mixed berries and honey

Lunch: Lentil soup with a side salad.

Dinner: Brown rice, mixed vegetables, and stir-fried tofu

DAY 3

Breakfast: Banana and almond butter rice cakes

Lunch: Quinoa stir-fried with turkey and vegetables.

Dinner: Baked chicken breast paired with asparagus and sweet potatoes

DAY 4:

Breakfast: Apple slices with cinnamon and oatmeal

Lunch: Omelet of spinach and mushrooms served with mixed berries on the side

Dinner: Stir-fried broccoli and beef over brown rice

DAY 5:

Breakfast: spinach, banana, almond milk, and chia seeds blended into a smoothie

Lunch: Quinoa salad with chopped tomatoes, corn, and black beans

Dinner: Grilled shrimp served with quinoa and steamed green beans

DAY 6

Breakfast: Scrambled eggs with garlic and sautéed kale

Lunch: Brown rice and skewered chicken and veggies

Dinner: Baked cod paired with roasted Brussels sprouts and a green salad

Breakfast: Cottage cheese with sliced peaches and honey drizzle

Lunch: Chicken breast with quinoa stuffed with spinach and mushrooms.

Dinner: Turkey and vegetable soup with mixed greens on the side.

Breakfast: Chia seed pudding paired with mixed berries

Lunch: Brown rice stir-fried with tofu and vegetables

Dinner: Wild rice and grilled fish with asparagus

Breakfast: Kale, pineapple, almond milk, and a dollop of protein powder combined in a smoothie

Lunch: Quinoa-based stir-fried veggies and lentils

Dinner: Curry of chicken and vegetables over brown rice

Breakfast: Apple slices and almond butter

Lunch: Omelet with spinach and mushrooms with a side salad

Dinner: baked chicken paired with green beans and sweet potato wedges

DAY 11:

Breakfast: Greek yogurt topped with sliced strawberries and honey drizzled over.

Lunch: Brown rice with veggie and turkey skewers for dinner

Dinner: Roasted Brussels sprouts and quinoa served with grilled shrimp

DAY 12:

Breakfast: Chopped tomatoes and spinach with scrambled eggs

Lunch: Lentil soup with a side salad.

Dinner: Steamed asparagus, baked fish, and mixed greens on the side

DAY 13:

Breakfast: Banana, spinach, almond milk, and chia seeds blended into a smoothie

Lunch: Quinoa curry with chicken and veggies

Dinner: Stir-fried broccoli and beef over brown rice

DAY 14:

Breakfast: Banana and almond butter rice cakes

Lunch: Mixed greens, bell peppers, and grilled chicken salad dressed with an olive oil vinaigrette

Dinner: Baked salmon served with quinoa and steamed broccoli

DAY 15:

Breakfast: Cottage cheese with mixed berries and honey drizzle

Lunch: Brown rice stir-fried with tofu and vegetables

Dinner: Turkey and vegetable soup with mixed greens on the side.

Breakfast: Apple slices with cinnamon and oatmeal.

Lunch: stuffed chicken breast with spinach and mushrooms and quinoa.

Dinner: Grilled fish served with wild rice and asparagus

Breakfast: Chia seed pudding paired with assorted fruit

Lunch: Omelet with spinach and mushrooms with a side salad

Dinner: Skewers of chicken and vegetables served with brown rice

Breakfasts: Kale, pineapple, almond milk, and a dollop of protein powder combined in a smoothie

Lunch: Quinoa-based stir-fried veggies and lentils for **Dinner:** Baked chicken paired with green beans and sweet potato wedges

Breakfast: Apple slices and almond butter

Lunch: Brown rice stir-fried with turkey and vegetables for dinner

Dinner: Roasted Brussels sprouts and quinoa served with grilled shrimp

Breakfast: Greek yogurt topped with sliced strawberries and honey drizzled over.

Lunch: omelet with spinach and mushrooms with a side salad

Dinner: Steamed asparagus, baked fish, and mixed greens on the side

Exercise Fitness and Lifestyle

A healthy lifestyle must include exercise, and those with B-positive blood types may find it helpful to customize their fitness regimen to suit their individual needs and interests. The following are recommendations for exercise for those who have blood type B:

A Balanced Approach: People who identify as B-positive typically benefit from a well-rounded fitness regimen that include bodyweight exercises, mind-body techniques, and cardiovascular activities like yoga and tai chi, as well as bodyweight and weight lifting workouts for strength training. Maintaining general health and fitness can be facilitated by this balance.

Take Note of Your Body: Observe your body's reaction to various forms of exercise. Adapt your regimen to your personal tastes, recuperation time, and energy levels.

Cardiovascular Activity: To strengthen your heart, increase your metabolism, and better handle stress, get regular cardiovascular exercise. Aim for at least 150 minutes per week, spaced out throughout the week, of moderate-intensity aerobic activity or 75 minutes of vigorous-intensity aerobic activity.

Strength Training: To develop and preserve muscle mass, incorporate strength training activities. Concentrate on full-body exercises that hit the main muscular groups. Try to get in two or three workouts a week.

Mind-Body Techniques: Yoga and tai chi are examples of mind-body exercises that can help lower stress and enhance flexibility and balance. These behaviors fit very nicely with the B-positive blood type diet's holistic philosophy.

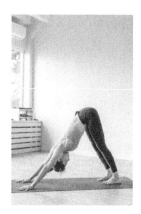

Outdoor Activities: Hiking, riding, and nature walks are among the outdoor activities that

B-positive people frequently take part in. Engaging in these activities offers a chance to improve wellbeing and establish a connection with nature.

Variety and Fun: Make sure your workouts are engaging and pleasurable. To keep yourself motivated and avoid getting bored with your workouts, try out some new sports, hobbies, or group exercise programs.

Keep Yourself Hydrated: Staying properly hydrated is essential for everyone, but B-positive people particularly need to remember this. Make sure you hydrate well prior to, during, and following your exercise.

Warm-Up and Cool-Down: Warm up your body before working out, and cool down to speed up recovery and lower your chance of injury after working out.

Speak with a Professional: A personal trainer or fitness professional can design a customized training program for you if you have special fitness objectives or health problems.

Keep in mind that your needs for exercise can vary depending on a number of personal factors, including age, fitness level, and any underlying medical issues. As such, it's critical to customize your workout regimen to your unique situation. For individualized advice on your workout regimen, always seek the advice of a healthcare provider or fitness specialist.

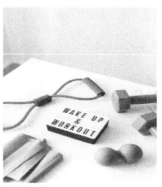

7-Days Meal Planner Timetable

DAYS	BREAKFAST	LUNCH	DINNER
SUNDAY			
MONDAY			
TUESDAY			
WEDNESDAY			
THURSDAY			
FRIDAY			
SATURDAY			

DAYS	BREAKFAST	LUNCH	DINNER
SUNDAY			
MONDAY			
TUESDAY			
WEDNESDAY			
THURSDAY			
FRIDAY			
SATURDAY			

Conclusion

To sum up, the Blood Type B-Positive Diet has been an empowering, transformative, and discovery experience. It's crucial to consider the most important lessons learned and the significant influence this unusual eating strategy can have on our lives as we get to the end of our investigation of it.

This book has proven to be an extensive resource for comprehending the ideas, foods, and way of life suggested by the Blood Type B-Positive Diet. We now know the science of the diet, the reasons behind matching our food preferences to our blood type, and the possible advantages it may have for our overall health and wellbeing. It has provided insights into how this customized strategy can assist us in reaching and maintaining a healthy weight, enhancing our mental clarity, improving digestion, and increasing our energy levels.

We've gone into great detail about what foods to eat and what not to, with an emphasis on whole grains, lean proteins, and certain fruits and vegetables. We have also discussed how to optimize the advantages of this eating plan by engaging in regular exercise, drinking plenty of water, and leading a balanced lifestyle.

As we've traveled, we've come across a plethora of mouthwatering and nourishing Blood Type B-Positive Diet recipes that offer a great culinary experience that suits our own dietary requirements and preferences.

In the end, this diet guide has provided us with a road map for changing our eating habits as well as a means of leading a better, livelier life. It has served as a reminder that we are in charge of our health, can make decisions that complement our own genetic make-up, and can benefit from a well-rounded, individualized approach to eating.

As we get to the end of this book, it is important to stress that being healthy on an individual basis is a journey with many facets and complexity, and the Blood Type B-Positive Diet is only one piece of the puzzle. It should be seen as an important tool that can help lead to a happier and more satisfying existence when used carefully and in concert with individualized healthcare guidance.

With the knowledge this book has provided, let's use it to make wise decisions, develop a closer relationship with our bodies, and keep moving toward our goals of achieving the best possible health and wellbeing. Recall that while blood type may serve as a foundation, what really matters is our dedication to living a healthier lifestyle and the decisions we make.

We appreciate you coming along for the ride. Cheers to accepting the Blood Type B-Positive Cookbook and all of its endless potential for a happier and healthier future.

If you enjoyed this book, kindly

leave a 5-star review on

Amazon.

Your wonderful review of this

book motivates me to continue

generating better work in the

future.]

Thank you very much!

Made in the USA
Las Vegas, NV
20 November 2024

12163253R00049